I HATE THE GYM

I HATE THE GYM

By Jessica Kaminsky

Illustrated by Sammy Yuen Jr.

SIMON SPOTLIGHT ENTERTAINMENT

New York London Toronto Sydney

SIMON SPOTLIGHT ENTERTAINMENT
An imprint of Simon & Schuster
1230 Avenue of the Americas, New York, New York 10020

SIMON SPOTLIGHT ENTERTAINMENT and
related logo are trademarks of Simon & Schuster, Inc.
Manufactured in the United States of America
First Edition 2 4 6 8 10 9 7 5 3 1
Library of Congress Cataloging-in-Publication Data

Kaminsky, Jessica.
I hate the gym / by Jessica Kaminsky ; illustrated by Sammy Yuen Jr.— 1st ed.
p. cm.
ISBN 0-689-87369-7
1. Exercise—Humor. 2. Gymnasiums—Humor. I. Title.
PN6231.E9.K36 2004
818'.607—dc22
2004011659

FOR ROCKY

I HATE THE GYM

CONTENTS

I believe every human has a finite number of heartbeats. I don't
intend to waste any of mine running around doing exercises.
—Neil Armstrong

J ust to clarify, this isn't a book about hating exercise.
Although I can't truly say it's a book about loving it either.
Rather, this is a book about a deeply complicated, borderline hostile relationship with a place I like to call . . . the origin
for all feelings of inadequacy. That's right, folks. We're talking
about the gym.

Most people have a love/hate affair with the gym. They
hate going but love the way they feel afterward; they love to
feel the burn. However, the relationship is never that simple.
When people truly dislike the gym, they don't just hate it—they
loathe it, despise it, and would rather swear off bread for all of
eternity than ever step foot in the place again. And yet these
admitted gym haters still drag their grumpy, hungry, tired
asses to the epicenter of evil. So the bigger question becomes
why; why do people go if they can't stand it? Because in the

heart of every gym hater lives the fear that, one day, they might become so obese that they will be restricted to wearing muumuus, loose-fitting track suits, or an oversized barrel for the rest of their lives.

Which brings me to this book. For years I dodged the gym like a sick friend during flu season. I even looked down on people with gym memberships. Not to mention, the idea of getting in a car and *driving* to exercise seemed totally absurd to me. I mean, why go to all that trouble when you could just put on your sneakers, open the door, and go? Which is what I did for years. I would jog around my neighborhood, watching as West Hollywood transformed itself from a crack-addled, hooker mecca (occasionally frequented by the likes of Hugh Grant) to a white picket fence, yuppie paradise. Look at me, I thought, not only am I working out, but also I'm simultaneously shopping for an adorable fixer-upper. And then later, when a friend gave me his old treadmill, I started jogging in the comfort of my own home. What could be better than watching the movie of my choice while exercising? Sadly, though, this was soon to change.

The truth is that even though I had been jogging for years, I never really noticed any physical change. I've always been skinny-to-smallish, depending on the time of year and my proximity to warm sesame bagels smothered in cream cheese. But I've never really been toned. I've always had leg muscles, but my arms were about as strong as a toddler's. It was embarrassing. So when my boyfriend and I got engaged and we started the exciting yet exhausting process of planning our wedding, I made a pact with myself to be the hottest bride I could be. And part of that was admitting that jogging alone wasn't going to cut it.

So, I, the original gym hater, joined a gym, got a trainer and, on my wedding day, was able to show off newly formed arm muscles. (Oh, and I have the pictures to prove it.) But I digress. The point is, I still hate the gym—the cheesy people, the funky smells, the sweaty equipment. But now, I know how to navigate it. That, and I finally found a gym where I always get a parking space.

CHAPTER ONE

INDUCTION

INTO THE CLUB

People who hate the gym tend to despise it passionately. They have strong visceral reactions—the techno music gives them a headache, the pungent smells make them nauseated, the lighting causes their eyelids to pulsate . . . which leads to the inevitable question: Could a brain tumor be far behind? And still, people force themselves to go to the gym. Why must we force ourselves to run on treadmills under florescent lights like lab rats in some cruel B. F. Skinner experiment? Whatever the answer, it's important to know your views on the matter. Are you an avowed gym hater, a gym tolerator, or an avid attendee? Which brings us to the quiz. How deep does your hatred run? And how far are you willing to go in order to never have to go back there?

Rate Your Hate: A Quiz

I. A trip to the gym makes . . .

A. your adrenaline surge and your heart rate leap. You just love to sweat and burn calories.

B. you want to put in overtime at the office. There must be a swamped intern around here who needs some extra help.

C. you want to break out a pint of ice cream and gorge yourself silly. The mere mention of the gym sparks a desire to consume fattening foods out of spite.

2. You receive a complimentary guest pass in the mail to a fancy gym around the corner from where you live. Your first reaction is to . . .

A. grab your duffel and head out the door. You'll take advantage of as many free passes as you can get.

B. make a spa day out of it, vowing to spend the entire time decompressing in the steam room.

C. crumple up the pass, toss it in the garbage, and wonder how the hell you got on that mailing list.

3. When a friend suggests you join them at the gym, you . . .

A. happily agree. It's been a decadent weekend of wine coolers, fish tacos, and Virginia Slims.

B. feign illness, claiming digestive turmoil brought on by questionable deli meats.

C. tell your "friend" to beat it. Clearly, this gym-loving goody-goody is no friend of yours.

4. You agree to be set up on a blind date by a coworker only to discover that the bachelor in question is a personal trainer. You . . .

A. can't believe your good luck. He's already way ahead of your last boyfriend, the dishwasher—not to mention the fact that his bod is bound to be a hunky slice of heaven.

B. try to look on the bright side: Dinner with a personal trainer could mean some free workout tips.

C. sit your coworker down and explain that, when it comes to men, you like them to at least have a fourth-grade minimum intelligence level, an ability to discuss something other than a high-impact workout, and preferably a beer gut.

5. If your gym burned to the ground, you would . . .

A. immediately run out and join another gym. You wouldn't want to fall behind in your workout. My god, think about what it could do to your stamina.

B. breathe a sigh of relief and celebrate this unexpected turn of events with a delicious, three-egg omelet.

C. hide the ski mask, oily rags, and gasoline tins. And start making some calls. You're going to need an airtight alibi.

6. You think of the people at the gym as your . . .

A. friends, buddies, pals.

B. partners in pain.

C. sworn enemies who must die.

7. **When someone gives you ten sessions with a trainer as a birthday gift, you . . .**
A. thank them profusely. This is the best gift ever.
B. can't help wondering if this isn't a thinly veiled hint to lose weight and firm up.
C. promptly try to hawk the sessions on eBay. Lord knows you won't be using them.

8. **You renew your gym membership every year because . . .**
A. the gym is like therapy. You need it to stay sane.
B. you'd be too ashamed *not* to renew it. In fact, you'd rather spend $800 on one aerobics class than admit you never go to the gym.
C. wait a second—you have a gym membership? When did that happen? You get enough exercise through sloppy sex.

Scoring:

A's = 1 point
B's = 2 points
C's = 3 points

8–13 points—**Avid Attendee:** Unless you're buying this book for an out-of-shape friend, you might want to reconsider the purchase. Because the results are in, and you don't even come close to hating the gym. In fact, you're what we call a gym-loving, personal trainer–lusting, health-conscious, calorie-counting, no-fun nerd. Not to get into name-calling. It's just, well . . . you may find some unkind words about people just like you written on the following pages. So consider this fair warning.

14–18 points—**Gym Tolerator:** You fall into the category of moderate to active gym hatred. It isn't high on your list of priorities, and yet you feel vaguely haunted by the fact that you haven't gone in three weeks. You wish you never had to go to the gym. But like many of us, you don't want to die of obesity at age forty. And osteoporosis applies to you now, not just to your grandmother. So sit back, pour yourself a glass of merlot, and enjoy this book. There is no shame in hating the gym. You are among the chosen people.

19–24 points—**Avowed Gym Hater:** How do I say this delicately? You're kind of scary. Your level of hate is on the extreme side. But then again, you are committed to hating the gym, and for that you should be recognized and applauded. It takes guts to fly in the face of the status quo. Just don't hurt anyone while you're at it.

CHAPTER TWO

MEMBERSHIP:

PENANCE FOR A FLABBY ASS

The End-of-the-Year Gym Membership Sale

The end-of-the-year gym membership sale is based on the principal that, in addition to laziness, people avoid the gym because it's too expensive. But the holidays have just come and gone, and there's no denying it: You've jumped pant sizes. So with the tantalizing "End of the Year" offer, how can you really say no? If you walk away from this, you are, in essence, turning down an opportunity to look hot. And you want to look hot, right?

This is exactly how they sucker you into a membership. . . . That's how they got me.

It was after the holidays, and I was feeling like a stuffed turkey. I'm not sure whether it was the second helping of pie or my inability to button my jeans, but I was vulnerable. And with New Year's Eve came New Year's resolutions and promises to be healthier, thinner, and generally more attractive to my partner.

And that's when the woman in the membership office spotted me. You know how they say dogs smell fear. Well, the folks in the membership office smell feelings of inadequacy. Within a matter of minutes I had bought a lifetime membership. I needed the gym, and they knew it. They had me exactly where they wanted me.

Pledge Week

Most salespeople work on commission. So when you roll into their office asking questions, they'll say whatever it takes for you to pull out your checkbook and sign up. If it's yoga you're interested in, they'll stress all of the different kinds of yoga—hatha, bikram, kundalini. They'll talk about the hot chai tea they offer on Wednesdays and the meditation spaces on the second floor. If you're into aerobics, they'll tell you about all the different types of high-impact classes they have on the schedule to accommodate your needs—cardio sculpt, boxerobics, power-step challenge. And if you're mainly interested in finding your next boyfriend, they'll tell you about the love connections that have been made at the gym. Whatever you need in a gym, they'll tell you they have it. They want new members and, more importantly, they want your commission. So if you let them, they'll keep talking, slowly beating you down until you have no choice but to pay to get rid of them.

So let's assume their sales pitch worked and you joined the gym. You will discover that, as a member, you'll receive a "gift package" that comes as a bonus when you sign up. The package usually includes: a body-fat analysis, a free session with a trainer, and gym passes for you to hand out to your other hopelessly out-of-shape friends in an attempt to peer-pressure them into joining as well. At first this seems like a magnanimous gesture. But beware the pseudo gift. This goody bag is designed to let you know . . . you need the gym.

Body-Fat Analysis

I recommend skipping the body-fat analysis entirely. But if you are a glutton for punishment and feel you must subject yourself to this kind of unique torture, my advice: Prepare for the worst. Most men have an average of 15 percent body fat, while women tend to come in slightly higher at 24 to 26 percent. This number is usually determined by a series of measurements and medieval fat-pinching techniques that are designed to embarrass you and make you regret the day you ever wore a bathing suit in public. Again, speaking from experience, I say pass on this offer. It's an exercise in humiliation that

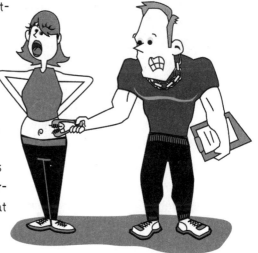

will leave you feeling depressed and housebound. So toss this mock present into the trash; there are some things better left unsaid.

Free Session with a Trainer

A free session with a trainer is yet another one of the thinly veiled pseudo gifts. So should you choose to use this "free session," remember your mother's words of wisdom: Nothing comes for free. Chances are your trainer will spend the bulk of your time together attempting to persuade you to sign up for more sessions. (Don't forget, the trainer is just another commission-hungry gym employee.) He will share no tips, no tricks of the trade, and no workout secrets. In fact, very little training and even less working out will occur. You probably won't even break a sweat. The session will consist of an hour-long sales pitch, with a detached, almost clinical, discussion as to why you need a trainer. Your body will be examined with an almost cruel lack of consideration. Your Buddha belly will be discussed. Your flabby arms (aka the "bingo wings") will be mentioned. And your thunderous thighs will be noted. Point being, your trainer will be mercenary in his attempts to bring you on as a full-time client. If this is something that you want and it will help you (which, of course, it can), then go for it. But don't give in if your trainer is creepy, sleazy, and reminds you of that horrible frat boy you once dated during freshmen year. Remember, you are spending a lot of money on this purchase, so don't let yourself be bullied. You want to get along with your future trainer. So ditch the meathead who makes you feel bad about yourself and go with someone you wouldn't mind spending an hour with.

Another tip when shopping for the right trainer . . . if you think he's pudgy or beyond beefy, don't sign up. Personally, I want my trainer (male or female) to have the kind of body that either I'd want or I'd want to be with. Some guy sporting a gut and a thick neck has no business training me. I certainly don't want to look like that. No, thanks.

Gym Passes

These complimentary passes are for you to distribute among your friends. And having been the recipient of several, they seem at first like a generous offer. You are allowed to use the gym, all of the equipment, the steam room, and the sauna as if you were a paying member. The idea behind these passes is that, once you use the facilities, you'll decide that you have to join. But you probably just want to use the gym for free. The thing is . . . they know this and will still try to do everything in their power to suck you in.

When I moved to Los Angeles, I was looking at a few different gyms when a friend told me about one around the corner from where I lived. It seemed ideal, albeit pricey. But the location was perfect, not to mention that I wouldn't have to drive and fight for parking (an ongoing thorn in my side). Armed with a guest pass, I entered the gym in question. But once my identity as a potential customer was discovered, I could not shake the lady from the membership office. First, she hijacked my driver's license, and then she insisted on giving me a tour, all the while forcing me to hear a sales pitch that lasted longer than most college lectures. By the time we were finished, I already felt like I had been through a workout. My head was tired from all the nodding, concentrated staring, and pretending to be interested. Finally, when I was able to get my ID back, I didn't want to exercise. All I wanted to do was flee. So if you decide to make use of the free guest pass, hang on to your ID and stand your ground.

Gym Cult(ure)

There are people who go to the gym every day for hours on end. They know the trainers' names, the woman at the front desk, the guy at the juice bar. They're down with the crew. In other words, they are the gym groupies. They train together. They eat alfalfa sprout sandwiches together. They share shots of wheatgrass, and spot one another in the weight room. This is NOT you. You have better things to do . . . like getting to know the names of the bartenders, the bouncers, and the cute guy at the dartboard. And that is okay. You are different. Always remember that. And different is better.

AWOL

Do you fear that swiping your underused membership card will trip a silent alarm, causing a personal trainer to descend on you like a used-car salesman? Have you not been to your gym in so long that it's a shock to learn they added a pool? Is your membership ID collecting cobwebs in your wallet? If so, you, my friend, are a delinquent gym member. You treat your membership like a needy child that you sponsor from a faraway land. In other words, it's something you do to make yourself feel better, and it doesn't hurt that it's also a tax write-off. Or perhaps you are the type of delinquent gym-goer who likes to keep your membership active out of guilt, in the hopes that one day you might be hit on the head and wake up a lover of exercise. But in truth, the last time you regularly went to the gym was during the Clinton administration. So, for god's sakes, stop pretending. This isn't school. You aren't going to get in trouble for poor attendance. You won't be sent to detention. So pocket the money and work on other, more worthwhile, things—like playing pool in dimly lit bars, making one-dollar jukebox selections, and honing your foosball technique.

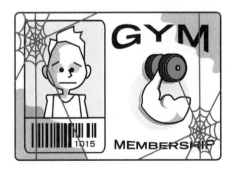

CHAPTER THREE

GETTING THERE:

THE FIRST HURDLE

Maybe you've blown the gym off all week. Or you haven't been in a month. Or worse, you can't remember the last time you used your membership card. Whatever the reason, it doesn't matter. The point is, you're there now. Well, at least you're imagining yourself at the gym, and that's one-sixteenth of the battle.

Many people don't realize that for the tried-and-true gym loather, the psychological battle begins before you even slip on your sneakers and head for the treadmill. Psyching yourself up to go to the gym after a hard day of work isn't easy; it often requires surmounting mental hurdles akin to climbing Mount Everest. The dread of knowing that your plans for the evening consist of being around sweaty people, bad lighting, and techno beats could dissuade even the most motivated person from going. That's when the impromptu no-carb diets commence and last-minute plans are made, all in an attempt to wiggle out of an evening of fitness. Because it's not simply about hating the gym, it's about the steely determination and sheer willpower it takes to overcome the first hurdle and drag our asses to a place we would do anything to avoid.

So the question is how to make the place we hate easier to deal with.

Set Goals

The key to easing the dread quotient of your workout is to set goals for yourself—reasonable goals. Like: If I go to the gym:

- I get dinner *and* dessert . . . and I'm not making it myself.
- I get one cocktail for every mile I run.
- I get to reward myself with an impulse buy.
- I get to eat as much chocolate as my belly can hold.

Another important device is to remind yourself why you're at the gym and what you're hoping to achieve.

- Do you want to make an ex jealous?
- Do you want to fit into your good-butt jeans?
- Is this punishment for a night of excessive drinking?

17

Whatever your motivation, having a specific goal in mind can really help focus a workout.

Remember the Half-Hour Rule

This rule may be obvious to the gym haters among you, but if you're at the gym for a half hour—it doesn't matter what you did—you worked out. It's like the "five-second rule," only you don't have to eat anything off the floor. Basically, the Half-Hour Rule allows you all the bragging rights you want. You can have a schvitz in the steam room, take a leisurely shower, and pamper yourself in the locker room. Because as long as you spend a full thirty minutes at the gym, you've passed the test. Now, pat yourself on the back and pick up a slice of pizza on the way home. Because today, you can honestly say you went to the gym.

Find a Gym Nemesis

This may sound strange to you, but I swear, it really helps take the sting out of a tedious workout: Find yourself a gym nemesis. Simply scan the crowd, lock in on someone totally annoying, and set about hating them like crazy for a good solid hour. By refocusing your hatred on an unsuspecting gym-goer, you'll release endorphins you never knew you had. Hate, after all, can be a strong motivator.

Another tip: You don't have to limit yourself to one nemesis. Collect an assortment of irritating characters to observe and mock silently. It can be "Crazy Dresser" one week, and "Slutty

Girl" the next. Your new nemeses will help you pass the time and ease the boredom of a workout. And let's face it, anyone who insists on wearing sunglasses while sweating on the elliptical machine is probably worthy of your hatred. One minute you'll be wondering what would ever possess someone to apply body glitter before going to yoga class, and next thing you know, your time is up and you've finished a half hour of cardio. See, having enemies can be a good thing.

Throw Money at the Problem

When I joined the gym, I did it because I was trying to look hot for my wedding. I wanted sleek, sexy muscles and impressive, picture-perfect abs. But I quickly discovered my biggest obstacle wasn't just the hard work it takes to get those things, it was simply waking up. I couldn't do it. And it didn't matter when I went to sleep or how rested I felt, the moment the alarm clock went off, I knew it meant peeling my sorry ass out of bed and tossing it onto a treadmill. I just couldn't rationalize putting myself through that. And so I slept. Which usually led to oversleeping. Which meant bed head at work and having to sustain comments from coworkers like, "You look different today. Did you get a haircut?"

So I devised a plan. I would set up several alarm clocks, each one beyond reach of the other. That way, I reasoned, I would have no choice but to get up and begin my day with a quick trip to the gym. But once the alarm went off, the snooze button was all too inviting, and inevitably I'd end up wasting a perfectly good hour of sleep by slapping the snooze button every ten minutes. And since it's hard to consider that exercise, although my wrist did feel sore, I realized the only way to solve this dilemma was to *throw money at the problem.* I had to pay for a trainer.

If I couldn't get myself out of bed, paying someone $60 to $100 an hour would definitely do the trick. I can promise you that the second cash is involved, you will not be late. It's an unspoken rule of self-preservation: When money is on the line, you will be on time. It's survival of the fittest . . . or the thinnest.

If you can't afford a trainer, or would rather spend the money on a decadent steak dinner and hearty Chianti, then take the more affordable approach and buddy up. The buddy system is certainly cheaper, and think of it as time to catch up on all the gossip with a friend while you exercise.

Here's what you do: Find a friend who loves going to the gym and get on their schedule. You might have to lie a little—make false declarations of love for the place you hate, or use some creative license when it comes to describing how often you go to the gym. Put yourself in your buddy's shoes—who would want to take on a lazy, deficient workout companion like you? But no matter. Charm your buddy. Coerce them into incorporating you into their workout regimen. If you agree to meet someone at the gym, then you know you'll go. You may be willing to let yourself down, but chances are you won't want to let yourself down in front of a friend.

Mix It Up

Mixing up your workouts is important. Because if you know exactly what you're about to put yourself through, you'll start to avoid going. That's what I did.

I once hired a personal trainer to design a workout for me. I couldn't afford to see him every week, so I asked him to show me a routine that I could do on my own. Sounds pretty smart, huh? That's what I thought. So my guy showed me this whole set of exercises that began with cardio, moved over to weights, then sit-ups, and eventually ended with some tension-band stuff and yoga-ball moves. It was great, everything I could've asked for. But when he wasn't standing next to me, my workout quickly devolved from impressive to adequate to eating bonbons in bed. And eventually any pretense of exercise was soon replaced by a long nap in front of the TV. That's when I realized not only did I need someone there to push me, but my dread stemmed from knowing that I had that same workout ahead of me every time. What I should have done was mix up my exercise routine into manageable chunks, but instead I was trying to do everything . . . which led to nothing. So, as they say, variety is the spice of life. Fight the boredom by keeping your gym experience interesting.

Fabricate a Gym Crush

Fabricating a gym crush is based on the same principle as finding a nemesis. Except in this case, replace the hate with lust. In other words, find a nice piece of eye candy, a hunky man or sexy lady to stare at and center some vague sexual fantasies around, and you'll be pleasantly surprised at how quickly the hour flies. Making up a gym crush to pass the time is a very effective distraction technique. Just go easy on the staring. No one likes a pervert.

Deal Breakers

You don't want to go to the gym—that's a given. But you force yourself to make the trip because your metabolism has slowed since college, and now it seems that everything you consume finds its way to your ever-expanding thighs. That said, there are some very legitimate reasons to prevent you from working out, some forces that are beyond your control.

For example, you're in the locker room, getting ready to work out, when you reach into your bag and you realize you forgot your gym lock. *Ding! Ding! Ding!* You just won yourself a "Get Out of Gym Free" card!

No gym lock = no workout. Think about it. You don't want to have to leave your bag, your wallet, your brand-new Juicy tee in an unlocked cubby, just begging for someone to steal them. Sure, you could always lug your giant workbag from the elliptical to the free weights, but that's a workout in and of itself. You're better off packing it in and trying again another time. But don't feel bad, you just got a *deal breaker*.

Deal breakers vary for each person. Mine are pretty straightforward. If I forget any one of the following items, I am free to turn around and leave the gym—no questions asked. In addition to forgetting the gym lock, my deal breakers are:

- **Headphones:** Part of being at the gym is being able to block it out. So no headphones, no deal.
- **Flip-flops:** If you have to shower at the gym, then you need flip-flops—this is nonnegotiable—preferably, the kind with the industrial-grade rubber soles that protect you from all kinds of gym slime. If you don't have the proper attire, you'll feel like you're barefoot in the employee bathroom at a triple-X theater.
- **Sneakers:** It seems obvious, but I've witnessed some adrenaline junkies exercising in boots.
- **Overcrowding:** This one is a little harder to determine. But there are times when you go to the gym and every piece of equipment is occupied. That's usually when I turn around and decide to leave. I can go again tomorrow. Life, after all, is too short to wait in line for a StairMaster.

CHAPTER FOUR

GETTING AROUND:

NAVIGATING THE MINEFIELD

Know Your Gym

The gym is like a minefield, chock full of sights, smells, and sounds you wish you had never witnessed. Like the guy in the stretching area doing lunges in short-shorts. Or the naked old lady powdering herself in the women's locker room. Or the man projectile-sweating in the weight room. That's why it's important to *know your gym*. Know it inside and out. Know where in the locker room the nudists congregate, where the nut jugglers hang out, and which is the fastest way for a quick exit. The better you know the place you hate, the more prepared you'll be for all of its curveballs.

Assess Your Comfort-ability

It took me a long time to feel remotely comfortable in the gym. Number one, I hated going, hence the book. Number two, I didn't know what the hell I was doing . . . hence the extreme pain and cramping that would follow any given gym visit. And number three, I often felt like Harrison Ford in *Witness*—a stranger living among strange people (spandex-clad beef cakes) with strange customs (grunting) and even stranger smells (body odor mixed with a spritz of Lysol.) The only difference is that, in the movie, Harrison Ford ends up bonding with the Amish and gets it on with Kelly McGillis, whereas I'd say at best there's a mutual tolerance between my gym and me.

I've always been easy to pick out at the gym. I'm the person studying the illustration on a piece of equipment, trying to decipher how to use it. This is then followed by an internal debate wherein I ask, "Do I really want bulging shoulders like the creepy man in the diagram?" And the answer is usually no, which shaves off a few good minutes of my workout.

Once I've finished having this discussion with myself, I head over to my other haunt, the elliptical machine, where I can be found concentrating hard at not falling off. This is probably the place where I feel most comfortable at the gym. Now, does that mean that I am truly at ease? No. Does my hatred of the gym still exist? Of course. Am I starting to sound like Robert Evans? You betcha. The point is, you just need to arm yourself with the necessary items (headphones, earplugs, mallet to crush meathead) to make your time at the fortress of evil a bit more tolerable. That and never stray into the weight room. But hey, you're the boss of you. Not me.

Locate Your Safety Zones

If you don't feel like you can relax (i.e., escape the man who keeps looking at you and scratching himself), then you won't want to work out. So whether your concern is lecherous looks from balding men or how to shake that creepy feeling of being watched while you're in the shower, it's important to remember: *Comfort is key*. And in order to truly feel comfortable at the gym, you need to create your own private, impenetrable workout bubble. So how do we achieve a sanctuary for ourselves within this hellhole? One word: buffers.

Buffers

A buffer by definition is a device used to cushion or reduce shock. And walking into the gym with all the lights, noises, smells, and scarring images can be a real shocker. So whether it's earphones to protect you from the blather (the Bubble Buffer), or working out with a friend (the Buddy Buffer), or hiring a trainer to keep you focused on yourself and not on the woman admiring her newly constructed breasts (the Bodybuilding Buffer)—buffers are essential to the easily distracted and easily disgusted gym-goer.

Adopt a Stance

Another approach is to think of the gym as a prison yard, or your own personal episode of *Oz*. Do you want people to feel it's okay to approach you? Or would you rather do your best impression of Christopher Lloyd on *Taxi* and be left alone? Assuming you'd choose the latter, I would suggest adopting a powerful scowl—or better yet, a mean, vacant stare. A well-timed scary look can strike the perfect balance between unapproachable and unpredictable.

Curious what effect this will have on your unsuspecting victim? Try one of these time-tested looks and watch in awe.

The Chief

If you're in need of character motivation, watch *One Flew Over the Cuckoo's Nest,* then pick your favorite character and imitate him. For instance, Chief really works for me. Remember, the stoic, stony faced, giant Native-American guy? Well, when I'm feeling watched, I just give a distant "I could smother you with a pillow" look, and it seems to work. Although I do recommend practicing in front of the mirror first—my first attempt at "the Chief" gave the general impression that I was suffering from constipation, and there's just nothing intimidating about that.

The Deranged Lunatic

If the Chief isn't your thing, then perhaps you should try this crowd pleaser—the Deranged Lunatic. Conjure up your most recent brush with that belligerent homeless man on your corner. At first, people might assume that you're talking passionately into your cell phone. But once they realize that in fact you're speaking to your dead cat, they'll give you all the space you need. Watch as the lines for the machines miraculously disappear.

The Recently Lobotomized

For those of you who have seen Jessica Lange's portrayal of the tragic Frances Farmer, you can incorporate some of her convincing moves into an even more convincing "Recently Lobotomized" look that is sure to keep people at bay. If you haven't seen that movie, then I recommend a smattering of head nodding, drooling, and giving someone a long, dead stare. This should keep the creepy people away because, frankly, you're the creepy one now. So once the coast is clear, sit back, settle in, and enjoy the peace and quiet. Now, if only they would stop playing that damn techno music. . . .

Mirror Abusers

The gym is a virtual fun house of mirrors. You can't turn a corner without being faced by one. Most gym-goers avoid them like an ex from a bad breakup, and take great pains to find the one machine out of the mirror's line of sight. Who the hell wants to watch themselves turn bright red and sweat profusely? Unless, of course, you're a certain buff, tan, handsome actor. My friend Aaron went to the gym one day and saw this guy standing in front of a triptych of mirrors doing arm curls, clearly enjoying the view. Let's call him Hasselhoff. Aaron secretly watched with a mixture of horror and awe. How could he and Hasselhoff even be considered part of the same species, let alone the same gender?

I think it's fair to say that anyone who relies heavily on

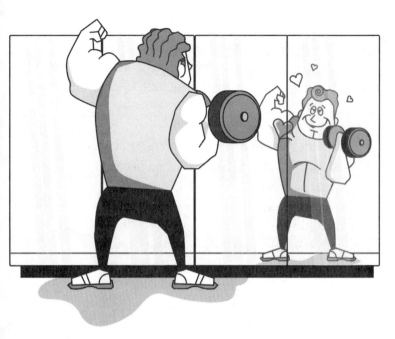

mirrors at the gym is enjoying the view. I, on the other hand, try my best to avoid the mirrors. For one, I don't need to see my butt from that angle. Not to mention, the mirrors are only going to show me what I already know: I am not a sexy sweater. Some women look flushed when they sweat, like they've just been embarrassed by an off-color comment, whereas I turn a deep purple. Think Violet Beauregarde after she eats the gumball. No exaggeration, I've had people come over and ask me if I'm all right, if I need water, if there's someone to call in case of emergency. That said, even if I were one of the chosen ones— the perfect sweaters—I still wouldn't be caught dead gazing at my reflection in the mirror. I'm at the gym to improve the view, not admire it. I hate the mirror abusers as much as I hate the gym. So get over yourselves and get back to work.

Noise Pollution

Noise pollution is one of the leading causes of gym hatred. So how do we deal with the bad music and the loud talkers? One word: headphones.

Headphones are essential for a pleasant gym experience (see Deal Breakers, page 22). They serve to protect and envelope your ears with familiar, comforting sounds. If you forget to bring them, I personally recommend immediate departure. However, if you are willing to brave the gym sans headphones, there are options for you. You can read a book or become engrossed in a magazine article. Although, let's be honest: Without the sound barrier, even the most compelling *Vanity Fair* article isn't going to drown out the girl loudly wondering to her friend why a guy she hooked up with hasn't called her back. Hmmm . . . I wonder why.

So what do you do when this happens? Personally, I like to cough loudly. It usually makes people think you're coming down with the flu or a case of whooping cough picked up from your last trip to the Ivory Coast. And trust me when I say this:

No one likes to be near a sick person. It's like getting on the red-eye and being seated next to a baby.

If the coughing doesn't get rid of the Loud Talker, try clearing your throat. And then keep clearing your throat. You'll either come off as incredibly rude and the oblivious Loud Talker will shoot you nasty looks as she continues to prattle on ad nauseum, or she will get the hint that you don't give a crap about her pathetic love life and she'll shut her trap. As far as I can see, it's a gamble worth taking.

Of course, it isn't always the Loud Talker's fault (as much as I hate to admit it). The problem usually begins with the overbearing music, compliments of the gym. Which in turn, causes a hideous ripple effect. Because now, the music is so loud that Loud Talkers have no choice but to talk even louder.

One way to deal with this problem is to cut it off at the source. You can walk into the office and complain to the management. But this is easier said than done for most people. Chances are, you'll feel ashamed for asking them to lower the music. What are you, ninety? Another way to go, if you have the time and inclination, is to write a strongly worded letter to the gym. Yes, it's dorky. But once it's on paper, it's official. And now it has to be dealt with. However, you could just save yourself some time and energy and bring your headphones. It's that simple.

CHAPTER FIVE

GYM ATTIRE:

LOWERING THE BAR, ONE OUTFIT AT A TIME

Dress for Sexxess

The idea of getting all dolled up for the gym is totally absurd to me. I mean, you're there to sweat, aren't you? Why would you want to wear something cute that you're just going to stink up? So girls, do yourselves a favor when changing for the gym: Save that sexy shirt and adorable pair of undies for a date. And go with the old T-shirt, loose sweats, and granny panties instead. Trust me, no one will be the wiser.

Although before I go any further, I must confess there's something I do when it comes to the gym that may seem slightly hypocritical. How do I put this without losing all credibility with my readers? I guess there's no way around it. I might as well just come clean. Fine, here it goes . . . I wear a thong while I work out. There, I said it. But before you get in a twist and start in on the name-calling, let me explain. I am a panty line Nazi. I'd hand out tickets to underwear offenders if I could.

That is how deep my disdain for the classic-cut pair of Jockeys runs. But rest assured, even though I work out in a thong, my G-string always remains discretely tucked beneath the waistband. Despite my love of the G, I hate when girls let their "whale tails" creep out of their pants—I'd give out citations for that offense, too, if I could. But this is my sickness. Not yours. So let's forget I ever mentioned it and move on.

Underwear aside, when I head to the gym, my look consists of an old T-shirt, or semiretired tank top (usually a staple that was once cute and is now either seriously stained or has lost its original shape), coupled with a pair of well-worn sweats. It's not a sexy look. I'm certainly not turning any heads. But then again, I'm not there to meet people. I am there to exercise . . . albeit reluctantly. But I still go. I mean, why else would I subject myself to this unique form of torture if I didn't want to look better? And why would I waste a good outfit on the gym?

In fact, most women I polled said they don't care what they wear to the gym. Many of them even admitted to purposefully *detracting* attention from themselves in order to go about their workouts free from smarmy stares and leering looks. For example, my friend Amanda contends that her hostility toward the gym runs so deep that she knowingly wears pants with holes in the butt. Not sexy bottom-baring holes like that Italian hottie in the movie *So Fine,* but tears and rips that send an overall message of disdain for the gym and the cheesy people in it. As Amanda put it, she has a lot of hate in her heart, and it's mainly directed at the perky girls and their perfectly coordinated outfits.

Unfortunately, scantily dressed girls are what we've come to expect at the gym. Without fail, anytime I catch a Bally's commercial on TV, I think I'm watching soft-core porn on Cinemax. Barely clad bodies glistening with hard-earned sweat, showing off yards and yards of legs and cleavage. And yet, if you think about it, it's a strange message to send: Come to the gym so you can look like this. Or, more accurately: Come to gym so you can watch people who look like this. Either way, gross. My friend Marni told me a story about how she forgot her exercise pants once and went to the gym boutique to buy another pair, when she discovered her only choices were either pink or blue. It's like forgetting your clothes for PE and having to put together an outfit from the lost-and-found box. Only, in this instance, it was as if her outfit were assembled by the sleazy director of a skin flick she didn't know she was starring in. Being a good sport, Marni wore the pink stretch pants only to discover after she had finished exercising that they were completely see-through and she had been flashing her bare ass to the entire gym. Oh, the horror.

Clothes Make the Man (or Woman)

A few women I interviewed confessed to giving extra thought to their workout outfits, as if a carefully put-together ensemble might help them do better in class. For instance, Dawn regularly attends a kickboxing class comprised primarily of gorgeous, perfectly toned and tanned women—essentially, extras from a Nike commercial. So before her class, Dawn finds herself carefully picking out her outfits, wanting to look as well groomed as her classmates. She contends that most of her attempts to fit in fashion-wise fail, which gives her extra motivation to push herself even harder in class. Fashion inferiority can be a powerful motivator.

While Dawn wants to blend in at the gym, my friend Aaron makes a point of looking like he doesn't fit in. When heading out to exercise, Aaron's attire usually consists of mismatched argyle socks, unfashionable shorts, and torn sneakers. By wearing this freaky combo, Aaron reasons that people will have lower expectations for him and his workout when they notice his unathletic getup. That way, he can surprise people with his unexpected strength. They'll say, "Wow, that bum is strong." Or at least, that's what he hopes.

And then there's my friend Ross, who doesn't think at all about what he wears to the gym . . . until he sees a sexy woman. That's when he remembers he's sporting a supernerdy improv shirt and realizes he's got no game.

In the end, it only seems to matter what you wear to the gym if you're looking to pick someone up or fraternize with the gym-loving in-crowd. If you fall into either of these two categories, we have a lot of work to do, my friend. Have I taught you nothing?

The Schlubby Hubby

Ahh, the schlubby hubby. You can spot him a mile away. He tends to wear rumpled shirts, rumpled shorts, rumpled everything, really. And he has that distinct "deer caught in the headlights" look about him, as if he's not sure whether to run on the treadmill or out the door. You see, the schlubby hubby is not your typical gym member. In fact, he thought that by getting married, he was exonerated from gym duty, not committed to a lifetime membership. But chances are, this taken man has been sent to the gym out of spousal mandate, or an attempt to drop the baby weight—that is, the sympathetic weight gain—that many a husband falls victim to during his wife's pregnancies. And now, they're exercising in a last-ditch effort to recapture the magic. But the truth is, you will never find a more sympathetic gym loather than the chubby hubby. One look in his eyes and you will see you've found a comrade. He abhors the gym deeply and despises the time he is forced to spend there. In other words, the schlubby hubby looks the way you feel. And for that, he demands your respect and friendship.

His favorite haunts: the stretching room, the steam room, and the sauna (i.e., any area requiring the minimum amount of exertion)
Likes: the moment his workout is over
Dislikes: knowing he'll be back the following day

The Bored Housewife

The bored housewife is a classic gym fixture. No matter what time you work out, be it rush hour or off-peak, she'll be there. She's the one dressed to the hilt, probably in something well coordinated and possibly cashmere. She's also in full makeup (another gym conundrum) with a rock on her finger that could wipe out hunger in most Third World countries. She can be found lounging by the comfy chairs in the lobby fielding calls on her cell phone.

In a sense, the gym is her office. Not that she ever really exercises or even sweats. If anything, she'll hire a hunky personal trainer to lift, flex, and stretch her leg for her. I mean, why push yourself when you can surgically alter your body and achieve the same results? The bored housewife is an interesting hybrid of dedicated yet indifferent.

Her favorite haunts: the lobby, the ladies' locker room, and the juice bar
Likes: attention from trainers
Dislikes: body odor and sticky surfaces

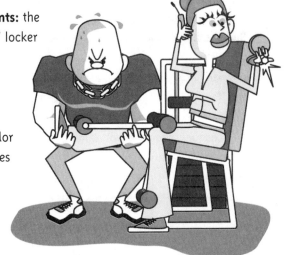

CHAPTER SIX

THE LADIES' LOCKER ROOM:
LETTIN' IT ALL HANG OUT

Navigating the Nudist Colony

The first time, as an adult, I was ever around a lot of naked women was during a spa visit with my mom. In addition to finding out what my tits are going to look like when I get older, I discovered just how many different types of women's bodies there are. Small boobs, giant cans, fake tits. Huge rump, tiny tush, no ass. Flat stomach, small tire, Buddha belly. And the list goes on. Now, transplant the same cornucopia of bodies into a smelly, unsanitary, cramped, crowded space where you wouldn't dare stand barefoot on the tile floor for fear of athlete's foot. And there you have it . . . the ladies' locker room.

The locker room is not unlike a subway car at rush hour—no room to move, dirty surfaces, and questionable characters. Like the subway, at times you have to contend with the hustle and bustle of pre- and post-work traffic. This involves bargaining for bench space, leg room, and locker access. While at other times during the day, the locker room is entirely free of crowds, which means you can take as much time as you need to put on your socks and brush your hair. Although given the fact that most locker rooms are unhygienic slime pits, I make it a policy to not linger. Why ruin a perfectly decent visit to the gym by accidentally stepping in something squishy? So, do yourself a favor and try to limit your contact with all locker room surfaces. And, above all else, do not put your bare bottom on a bench. My god, woman, have some decency. Do you want to catch a rash?

And finally, just like a subway ride, no trip is complete without an interaction with a lunatic. Whether it's the old lady talking to herself or the bimbo on her cell phone, it's tough not to stop, stare, and listen. But do yourself a favor; as much as you'd like to gape, put your head down and keep moving . . . unless you want to tangle with the woman tweezing her mustache. But my guess is, you don't, which is wise. So get in and get out to limit contact with germs and crazies.

There's a Fungus Among Us

Showering with flip-flops is nonnegotiable. I can barely touch my bare foot to the ground without feeling like I've become a breeding ground for disease. Which is why industrial-strength flip-flops are a must. In addition to protecting your feet from fungus, thick flops ward against unpleasant encounters with detritus like tumbleweed-size hairballs and errant hairs. To shower without them would be like having sex with Colin Farrell without a condom. And let's face it, that's just not smart.

Locker Blockers

Without fail, anytime I'm in a rush there is someone parked right in front of my locker with the entire contents of their gym bag spread out on the bench like it's their suite at the Four

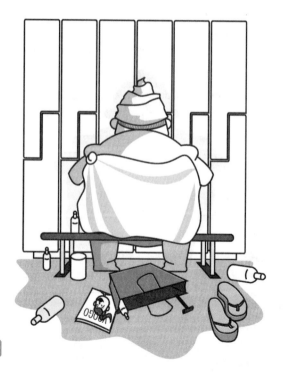

Seasons. It's the Murphy's Law of the locker room: No matter how many empty lockers there are, someone will always end up in the one right next to yours. So once you've squeezed into position next to your locker, you can now begin the difficult task of getting dressed. This involves an awkward naked balancing act, contorting your body so as to expose the least offensive view to your neighbor, all the while negotiating your towel coverage as you try to put your jeans and bra on without flashing your breasts to the world.

So, how do you deal with the sedentary set?

1. Master the art of the quick change.
- Begin by drying off in the shower so as to reduce the time spent toweling off in cramped quarters.
- Organize your clothes so that they're in the order in which you'll put them on (i.e., underwear on top, then shirt, pants, etc.)
- In a pinch, lose the bra. This saves time and energy.

2. Relocation, relocation, relocation!
- If you are in need of a little extra elbow room and the Locker Blockers are cramping your style, don't be afraid to pick your stuff up and move.
- Too many looky-loos? Remember, you can always change in one of the bathroom stalls.

3. Screw it!
- Just change at home.

Nude Encounters of the Weird Kind

One of the more uncomfortable locker room experiences is the stark-naked run-in with someone you barely know. Whether you're emerging from a shower or putting on your clothes, do not be surprised when you come face-to-face with someone you either just met or haven't seen in years. This is usually followed by an utterly awkward silence as you scramble for conversation and your underwear at the same time. The first time it happened to me, I chalked it up to bad timing. But when I ran into another person I hardly knew while I was naked, I started to detect a trend. It might not be discussed publicly, but nude encounters happen all the time. So don't be surprised the next time you see your boss trying to wrangle her sports bra on as you struggle to pull up your underwear under a towel.

The Scales: Obsessive Weighers

Women get crazy about their weight, and never has that insanity been more pronounced than in the ladies' locker room. At the center of this obsession is the scale—not one of those inaccurate, off-by-five-pounds bathroom scales, but a professional, chillingly exact, doctor's office scale.

Naked women, young and old, of all shapes and sizes, march up to it one by one to see if they've miraculously shed all of their unwanted weight in a single hour at the gym. Within this group there are a few different kinds of weighers:

• **The Loud and Proud:** These are the particularly annoying breed of women who weigh themselves and then proudly step off the scale, leaving their new weight for all the world to admire. Just remember, it's not wrong to hate these women . . . nor is it wrong to want to tie them down and force them to eat doughnuts.

• **The Weight Watchers:** After removing any item (watch, bracelet, contact lenses) that might minutely alter their weight, these women sheepishly approach the scale as if it might give them an electric shock for gaining a pound. Once on the scale, they maneuver the weights nervously and then leap off and return the scale to zero, removing all evidence of said weight gain or loss.

• **The Naked Weighers:** These are the people who insist on being stark naked when weighing themselves. As if the one eighth of an ounce in bra and panty weight will tip the scale. You can only imagine these are the same people who read labels, count calories, and measure the fat content of their food. As far as I'm concerned, that's no way to live.

My advice is to ignore the scale entirely. Instead, go by how you feel, how you look, and how your clothes fit. I can always tell whether I've lost weight by the way my jeans feel. Are they tight around the butt? Is the bottom baggy? Do I have to undo the top button after dinner? These are the signs of weight fluctuation. But they're normal, so don't freak out. And if you're smart, you'll stay the hell away from the scale.

Mirror Hogs

The name says it all. Mirror hogs are those irritating people who spend too much time plucking their eyebrows, examining their pores, and applying makeup at the gym. No matter what corner of the mirror you may need to use, they block your view. At first, you try to move around them, politely clearing your throat once then twice to indicate that you, too, would like to put on some makeup. But these signals don't mean anything to the mirror hog. She is immune to your amateur technique. Most mirror abusers are pushy by nature, so if you would prefer to not tussle with them, you can either turn to the mini mirror in your compact or alter your schedule to avoid this recurring issue.

That said, there is a distinct difference between the morning, evening, and lunchtime rush-hour crowds. The before-work exerciser approaches the mirror in a methodical, efficient, all-business style; the after-work exerciser takes her time in front of the mirror as if nursing an invisible cocktail; and the lunch hour exerciser falls somewhere between hurrying to get back to the office yet reluctantly dragging her feet. Whatever the hour, it's annoying to be unable to sneak a peek at your reflection. So either confront the narcissist head on or go to the gym at odd hours.

Ladies' Locker Room Etiquette

People treat the locker room like it's their personal bathroom. They clip toenails, clean hair brushes, and leave dirty Q-tips on the counter. This is not acceptable. The rules of conduct are very simple:

- Keep it clean.
- Be respectful.
- Don't linger.
- You soil it, you boil it.

The Players

The Seniors: They come to the gym most days for low-impact exercise (usually water aerobics) and human contact. Interestingly enough, for folks who consider their time precious, they certainly spend a lot of it dawdling in the locker room, gabbing loudly. The seniors are, for the most part, sweet and benign, but as a group they fail when it comes to regard for others.

Consideration Rating: 5.5

The Housewives: Chances are, they find the locker room as unpleasant as you do; however, for them, a trip to the gym is a day off. There are no kids tugging on their sleeves, no counters to clean, and no laundry to fold. Which is why, for this group, the locker room is just another sniveling child—messy, sticky, and in need of a scrubbing. And for that reason, the housewives refuse to spend excessive amounts of time in the locker room. They are not your biggest problem.

Consideration Rating: 8

The Exhibitionist: Known for keeping their breasts out as long as possible, the exhibitionists are the ones doing gynecological stretches in the locker room and toweling themselves off as if moisture were a punishable offense. Exhibitionists can be young or old, short or fat, tall or skinny. The only thing that unites them is their desire to be naked and stay naked. They are a breed unto themselves.

Consideration Rating: 1

CHAPTER SEVEN

THE MEN'S LOCKER ROOM: VALLEY OF THE BALLS

Cock of the Walk

Before we get into a lively discussion of the men's locker room, I must confess that this is the one place in the gym I could never gain access to despite numerous (denied) requests. For obvious reasons, of course. So instead, I turned to my male friends and after doing countless interviews, I was able to put together a rather full picture of what goes on behind closed doors through their collective experience in the locker room.

For starters, like the ladies' locker room, nudity is in abundance. There are loungers, saunterers, proud peacocks. Air driers, towel driers, drip driers. There's the proud exhibitionist, who struts around with the least amount of clothes possible, and the shy hibernator, who cowers in the corner like a late bloomer in a junior high school locker room. In fact, almost every man I spoke to confessed that their gym experience would improve significantly if they could avoid the men's locker room. Which leads to the question: If the locker room experience is so jarring, then why not just skip it entirely? Well, the problem is, most men need to use the locker room. They have jobs to get ready for in the morning and people to meet after work. And while they might not be one of the loud and proud nudists, they still need to use the shower, shave, and change. So read on, fellas, and find a useful tip or two on how to fend off unwanted stares and steer clear of the wet spot.

Size Matters

Straight boys, beware: Sexual preference can be determined by the size of your toiletry bag. The bigger the bag, the gayer the lad.

As my friend Johnny explained to me, you can always spot the straight boys. They're the ones quickly applying the Right Guard deodorant under their shirts and then dashing out the door. Whereas the gay boys are prone to primp. They usually have toiletry bags that could rival those of the most high-maintenance sorority girls. They have their shampoos and conditioners, tweezers and trimmers, scrubs and creams.

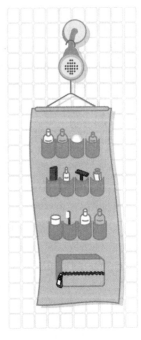

So boys, when you're packing your morning kit, remember size does matter. Consider yourself warned.

Shower Hour

From what I've gathered, there are a variety of different types of showers in the men's locker room. There's the "group shower" with different shower heads positioned around the room, which is reminiscent of high school. And then there's the individual shower stall both with and without shower curtains. Obviously, the showers with curtains are the most civilized and therefore the most coveted; unlike the showers with no curtains, which leave the bather with the vague sense of being a participant in an Amsterdam peep show.

Basically, everyone I spoke to, both gay and straight, said that the showers always have a slightly menacing vibe, leaving the person to feel like they're always on display. And for this reason, the shower experience often becomes a race against the clock. Your goal: to wash and dry as quickly as humanly possible. But before you even commence cleaning, pole position is key. My friend Chris feels it's important to stake out a corner of the shower so, as he puts it, "you're protected on both sides." Whereas Ross prefers to take what he calls a "defensive stance" by facing out of his shower stall, never surrendering his rear. The overall consensus seems to be that the shower is never relaxing, and while you may leave cleaner than when you first arrived, you're always rushing to finish. And, chances are, you probably still have some soap behind the ears.

Shave It for a Rainy Day

To shave or not to shave, that is the question. And the answer is, if you can hold off, give your razor a rest.

As someone who has lived with a beard-shaving male for several years, I can tell you, hair is a pain in the ass. It gets clogged in drains, caught in tiles, and stuck on soap. And it doesn't stop there. Hair is seemingly easy to spot but is small in length and hard to gather. In other words, hair goes everywhere. And no matter how many times your guy claims to have cleaned up the bathroom, beard trimmings have a way of reappearing minutes later. They're the cockroaches of the grooming world. So before you shave, think of your fellow gym members and the underpaid maintenance staff who will inevitably be stuck battling the hairy aftermath, and save the shave for another day.

Avoiding Germs

Unless your plan is to seal yourself in a full-body condom, you will be battling sticky surfaces, dirty tissues, and the inexplicable wet spot. So keep your hands clean, the antibacterial soap flowing, and your flips-flops within arms reach. If you treat the locker room as you would a contaminated area (think Cher in *Silkwood*), you should be able to keep germs at bay.

When using the showers, always be sure to wear flip-flops. Showers are a fungus fest. The less you touch, the better. In fact, to be safe, you might even need to shower after the gym shower. It's your call. All I know is, there's a fine line between athlete's foot and stinky foot.

Of course, for the true germaphobe, there are other precautions that can be taken in your quest for a slime-free existence:

- Don't touch skin to surface.
- Avoid the manhandled handles—open doors with a paper towel.
- Mind the wet spot.
- If it's yellow, bellow.
- If there's an issue, use a tissue.
- Play it safe: Avoid the men's locker room altogether and shower at home.

Men's Locker Room Etiquette

When venturing into the locker room it is essential to know what to do, where to go, and how to protect yourself, which is why an understanding of etiquette is a must to thrive and survive.

- Don't drop your soap in the shower.
- Don't forget your flip-flops.
- Don't let your eyes wander.
- Don't crowd your neighbor.
- Don't towel-dry your balls.
- Don't linger in the locker room.

The Players

The Macho Man: He's the cartoonish-looking guy with the giant neck and bulging arm muscles, and the teeny-tiny legs that make him look like he could tip over at any time. These men are always at the gym no matter what the hour or the holiday. While they may be physically intimidating, they have no interest in you . . . other than to bench-press you for fun. Their love affair is with the free weights, not your scrawny ass.

Threat Rating: 2

The Peeper: He's the guy who gives you that unsettling feeling that you're always being watched. But don't worry—he won't make a move. He's a peeper. And though he may not be the type to cross the room for a chat, like it or not, he'll be thinking about you later.

Threat Rating: 3

The Creeper: He stares too long. He stands too close. And if he sees an opening, he'll come over and talk to you, using such winning lines as, "Has anyone ever told you that you look exactly like Kevin Bacon?" So don't give him an opening, and travel in pairs whenever possible.

Threat Rating: 5

The Hairy Guy: The name says it all. He's the unfortunate fellow sporting a suit of hair. His body screams, "Wax me." He's so hairy that if he was naked in the woods, he'd be in danger of getting shot by a hunter. Best to just look away and thank god you're not him.

Threat Rating: 0

The Poser: He's the guy who is in love with his physique. He's usually found strolling around the locker room naked. In fact, he prefers to do everything naked. He shaves naked. He blow-dries his hair naked. He flexes his muscles in front of the mirror naked. In other words, he is head over heels madly in love with himself. And you're just getting in the way of the love affair. So step aside.

Threat Rating: 1

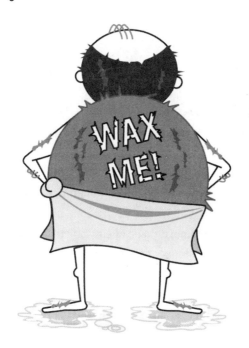

CHAPTER EIGHT

THE FITNESS ROOM:
WIPE IT DOWN

Have you ever had the delightful experience of getting on a machine only to find yourself covered in another person's sweat? If your answer is yes, you're not alone. Inconsiderate sweaters lurk everywhere. They're obliviously getting on and off equipment all over the gym. And the last thing you want is to be left with a towel drenched in someone else's sweat. So how do we handle this cadre of thoughtless workout fiends?

Here's a tip: When you see someone getting ready to leave behind an overly moist piece of equipment, try tapping him on the shoulder (although he's probably covered in sweat, so a simple "Hey, you!" will suffice) and saying, "I think you forgot to take care of something." This should do the trick. And even though "sweaters" aren't known for their considerate behavior, shaming them into action should work—just be prepared to stand your ground.

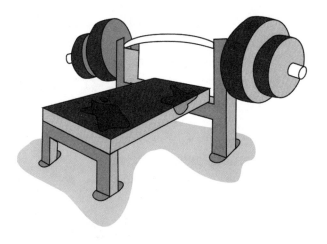

Sweatin' to the Oldies

Every gym has one—the oblivious workout queen. She sings to the music, waves her arms in the air, and moves her butt to the beat. She makes you feel embarrassed, and you don't even know who she is. She's like someone's drunk, inappropriate aunt. In fact, with all of her prancing around, it's surprising she's even able to stay on course on the treadmill. But miraculously, she does. And as long as she doesn't catch you, it's always good for a laugh to watch and make fun of her.

And where there's a workout queen, there must also be a king. He's the man in the seventies-era tracksuit and headband who farts loudly and often. He may make you nostalgic for your grandpop. But beware, it's the old guys who often are the secret perverts of the gym. My friend Amanda was watching a group of older men suiting up for a game of racquetball. She smiled and said hi. And as she walked past, she heard one of them say, "Nice ass, sweetheart." She couldn't believe her ears.

Running as Fast as I Can

I've been running for years; first on the cross-country team in high school, then around my neighborhood, and most recently, on the treadmill at the gym. I run an average of two to three miles, depending on how fat I feel and how close I am to bathing suit season. And yet I have never once come close to achieving the coveted "runner's high." I hate running. Some days, I can distract myself by reliving a frustrating work encounter or by watching a funny episode of *Seinfeld* on the gym television. But most days, it's hell. And I've never come close to a state of euphoria . . . unless by euphoria we're talking sheer exhaustion and pain.

I think it's time to debunk the myth. The "runner's high" (or rather, lie) is a concept put forth by the sneakers companies in order to get people to run longer and faster, thus causing their sneakers to wear out sooner. Of course, this is an unproven theory. But I'm pretty sure I'm onto something.

Abusing the Rules

In almost every gym I've visited (and I've logged in a lot of time at many mediocre gyms), there are signs posted around the cardio equipment (treadmill, elliptical machine, stationary bike, etc.) asking members to be considerate and only use the machines for thirty minutes during peak hours. And yet, almost everyone abuses this rule. People don't care if someone is waiting. They probably had to wait themselves, so why should they abide by the rules when the person before them didn't? And so the cycle of thoughtless gym behavior continues. To this I say, it must end! Hitching up the ass-wagon and dragging it to the gym is tough enough to begin with, but having to wait in line to use a piece of equipment is torture. If you see someone waiting, be a sport and stick to the rules.

Fitness Room Etiquette

If this were a perfect world, all gym members would abide by a reasonable code of polite conduct. Imagine a world where you set the rules and read on:

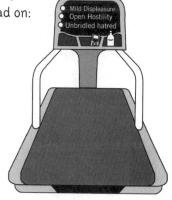

Mild Displeasure
Open Hostility
Unbridled hatred

- Wipe down your machine.
- Keep the farting to a minimum.
- Bring headphones to drown out neighboring grunters.
- Don't sing out loud. This isn't a karaoke bar.

The Players

The Anorexic: She's the one who's unsettlingly thin and is working out harder than everyone else. She's at the gym so often, you're starting to think she lives there.

Your Goal: Get out of the way before her toothpick-thin legs snap and she flies off the treadmill.

Mr. Midlife Crisis: He's in the process of trying to recapture his youth and his physique. He sports the newest in fitness gear. His hair is dyed, his nails manicured, his soul empty.

Your Goal: Run like the wind to avoid the suffocating wafts of Drakkar Noir emanating from his sweaty body.

The Gay Man: He lives and dies by his workout. He spends more time at the gym than at his job. And it isn't uncommon to find him working out in designer threads. Style matters to this one. And chances are, he's going from the gym to the club.

Your Goal: Let this workout queen be . . . unless you have someone to set him up with.

The Old Man: He's there under doctor's orders and is desperately trying to prevent his second heart attack. He sweats profusely and appears to be in great pain. Stand back and give the geezer some room to breathe. You don't want him dying on your watch.

Your Goal: To be far away when he has his next cardiac arrest.

CHAPTER NINE

THE WEIGHT ROOM:
MUCH ADO ABOUT NAUTILUS

Venice Beach Meets Prison Yard

If you've ever spent any time in the weight room at the gym, you know it can be very intimidating. Not only do people barely speak to one another, but everyone seems to know exactly what they're doing. It's like synchronized swimming for beefcakes.

Watching the antics of the weight room is a primeval experience. Man spots weight. Man approaches weight. Man lifts weight. Man grunts and lifts again. In short: Lift, grunt, repeat. Or in the event of two dudes working out together, it's lift, spot, grunt, repeat. The result of these weighty exercises is bigger muscles at the cost of a thicker neck. That's right, along with the growing pecs come bulging veins and an ever-widening neck. But please, continue. Lift, grunt, repeat. Don't mind me. I'm just going to take my five-pound weights for a little walk.

No (Wo)man Zone

One thing you might notice upon entering the weight room (other than feeling uncomfortable and a strong sense of not belonging) is that it is a sea of men. Guys are wordlessly spotting, lifting, and grunting. And there isn't a female to be found. Well, there may be one or two adventurous souls. But they're just as unapproachable as the men. The most intimidating part of the weight room is that everyone knows exactly what they're doing. They have a routine, and they have it down pat. They understand the politics and the etiquette, and they execute their routines with military precision.

When I first entered the forbidden zone, I made some classic rookie errors. I interrupted two workouts and accidentally cut in on someone's "set." I was a walking disaster. But I couldn't just turn around and leave. If I was ever going to achieve the desired tricep arm muscle (part of the hottest-bride-to-be program), I needed to know what weights to use and how to use them. And so I decided to bust out the big guns—enter my trainer, Rob.

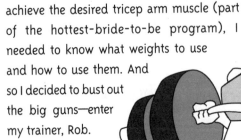

Rob walked into the weight room with the confident swagger of a man who intimately knew his weights. He showed me where to go, what to use, and which mirror to stand in front of. And then, he stood back as I completed my set of curls. And for the first time, I was lifting, grunting, and lifting again. Just like the big boys with the prison tattoos. At last, I fit in. Well, sort of. I lacked the bulging veins and Popeye muscles, but I felt confident that I could get there if I wanted to.

A word to the wise: Hire a trainer for your first trip in. Or get a knowledgeable friend to escort you into the weight room and show you the ropes. You need to know which weights to use and which to avoid. And while you may never have that self-assured trainer strut, at least you'll know you're one curl closer to beautifully toned arms.

Spotters

Granted, bench pressing is not my thing. But in asking around, I discovered that spotting and "spotting etiquette" seem to be the hot-button issue among the boys.

From what I gather, the concerns seem to be threefold. There are the people who need a spot and get attitude for asking. There are the people who offer to give a hand and then spot incorrectly. And finally, there are the people who agree to spot and don't pay attention as the lifter struggles beneath them. Like the story my friend Ross told me about bench pressing with a spotter when an earthquake hit. The spotter dashed out, leaving Ross pinned under the weights, until the guy came to his senses and returned to free him.

Push, Push in the Tush

Lifters beware: Everyone's farting up a storm in the weight room. I mean, what do you expect? When you're squeezing, grunting, and pushing, the occasional gas leak is bound to happen. Here are some tips to guard against such toxic spills and malodorous scents:

- While spending time in the weight room, switch to mouth breathing.
- Bury your nose in your shirt. Your own stink is better than the dude's next to you.
- Keep it quick. Don't dillydally.
- Remember, you can always do weights tomorrow.

Weight Room Etiquette

If there's one place in the gym where it's vital to observe proper etiquette, it's the weight room. With the amount of testosterone coursing through the room, considerate behavior (unless you want to tangle with one of the big boys) is more than mandatory. So pay attention:

- For the love of god, don't bang your weights together.
- Don't fart freely.
- Wipe down your bench after you use it. No one wants to sit in your sweat.
- Put your weights back when you're done.
- Don't shout while you're lifting. It's alarming and distracting.

The Players

The Steroid Guy: The vein in his neck is throbbing, and he looks like he might snap and punch someone in the face at any time. He's your classic rager. He's serious about his workout, and he doesn't want anyone getting in his way. So trust your instincts and move. He's a live wire.

Your Goal: Avoid the 'roid.

The Mirror Man: The name says it all. He likes to work out in front of the mirror, preferably with his shirt off. He's interested in one person and one person only: himself. And he feels compelled to monitor his muscle development with every curl—even if it means blocking your access to the weights.

Your Goal: Get him to move.

The Stinkers: They're the guys who roll out of bed and head straight for the gym. They have horrible breath and rank body odor. Unfortunately, they're usually the ones working out the hardest, detonating their stink bombs for all to suffer through. So either commence mouth breathing, or clear the area.

Your Goal: Shake the stench maker.

The Yeller: He's the guy who lifts and lifts loudly. Like Monica Seles on anabolic steroids, he's working hard and he wants you to know it. So do your hearing a favor and stay one step ahead, or suffer the ear-shattering consequences.

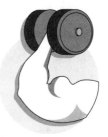

Your Goal: Protect your eardrums.

CHAPTER TEN

THE CLASSES:
HIGH SCHOOL REVISITED

It doesn't matter which class you choose. Spinning, step, or yoga, exercise classes are like being back in school all over again.

For starters, the dynamic is the same. You have a teacher who stands in front of a bunch of students who are there to learn. The teacher shows everyone the moves; the class awkwardly attempts to follow along. Some pick it up with ease, while others stumble through the motions. At best, it's an hour of solid sweat. At worst, it's an exercise in humiliation, immediately followed by vows of never returning. But how, you might ask, could an exercise class cause such emotional turmoil? The question can be answered in three simple words: high school revisited.

It's the cool kid versus the geek, the jock versus the spaz, and so on. Exercise classes, like high school, have a unique and intense caste system that could rival any Hindu society. There are the "teacher's pets" (the dorks and future leaders of the world who like to be front-and-center, eager to learn every step, lunge, and kick); the "slow learners" (the seniors, and, let's be honest, sometimes me); the "class clowns" (the uncoordinated women who deflect with humor, also me); the "beginners" (the husbands forced to attend by their wives); the "shy nerds" (the poor souls who lack the self-esteem to move their bodies comfortably); the "rebels" (the men and women who find their teacher odious and wish they were somewhere, anywhere else); and the "outcasts" (the folks who attend class so infrequently, it's always brand new to them).

No matter what category you fall into, it's always fascinating how seriously people take the classes. From the placement of their yoga mats to arriving early enough to secure a favorite set of weights, classes bring out the inner bitch in all of us, and can be so much more than physically challenging. They are both a lesson in restraint and in asserting oneself. No matter what it is, a class is survival of the fittest—and the quickest.

Boot Camp

I attended several "boot camp" classes, which live up to their name with their militaristic drills and punishing exercise techniques. Boot camp was an hour-long class that promised "challenging options for athletic conditioning through calisthenic drills" and boasted that it would "push you to the limit." And did it ever. I spent the next day hobbling around, easing myself in and out of chairs.

The first thing the instructor did was divide the class into five groups. Each group had a different workout task. There were two arm-curl stations, an area to do sit-ups, a corner dedicated to jumping jacks, and then the cruelest drill of all: wind sprints. Remember those from PE—or have you blocked them out?

Within two rotations, I knew that by the time the sun came up the next day, I wouldn't be able to walk, move, or even lift my arm to beckon for help. I was in major trouble. And there was not a bath in the world that could reverse the imminent pain. But the worst part of the class came when the teacher told us to run around the room, and then threw balls at us to test our reflexes. Could this really have been part of the class, or were we being punished for Sarge's bad day? As the balls continued to fly at our heads, I began to think the latter, and marshaled my remaining strength to duck, dodge, and avoid the missiles. Finally, when boot camp was declared over, I slowly limped to the teacher and informed him that he had crippled me. He nodded and smiled, clearly pleased with what he took to be an endorsement of his teaching skills. "No, you jackass!" I wanted to shout. "That's not a good thing. I wasn't complimenting you. I was criticizing you." So if you're nostalgic for the days of PE and abusive, power-hungry teachers, then "boot camp" is the place for you. Otherwise, steer clear. And remember: You're not going to be held back a year if you fail to show up. Thankfully, those days are far behind you.

Spinning—Out of Control

One might think that people who love "spinning" love biking, and by extension, love nature. Right? Wrong. Spinning and real cycling have nothing to do with each other. Spinners are not lovers of nature. They are lovers of their bodies, their abs, and their perfect butts. They are working actors, wanna-be actors, and all-around narcissists. They are obsessed with how they look and what it'll take to look even better. And spinning, which is an hour of sheer hell, is the most twisted way to achieve this goal. It is the ultimate "type-A" workout. It's an intense, total body sweat-a-thon.

So having spent my whole life avoiding this exact type of exercise, I decided to give it a chance and accompany my friend Kristen, an exercise fiend, to one of her spinning classes. First thing I learned was, don't get in the way of a spinner and her bike. It's like separating a Doberman from raw meat, or me from a glass of wine—very dangerous. It became clear that, in the world of spinning, getting the right bike is everything. Kristen explained that the front row was reserved for the diehards and regular attendees. Had I nabbed one of the coveted front-row bikes, I would have had to prove to the instructor and the class that I was the new top dog. And since I hadn't been on a bike in over five years, that would have been tricky. Wisely, I took a seat in the last row, free from ridicule.

As promised, the class was an unbridled nightmare. Twice, I thought I might die. I sweated more in forty minutes than I ever had in a lifetime. In fact, I learned that my ears can and do sweat. Not to mention, because this was my first time in the class, I didn't know to bring my own, cushiony bike seat. So when the class was through and all of the perfect people hopped off their padded seats, I went home with a chafed ass that a day later blossomed into a giant butt bruise. Let's just say that I won't be returning. Spinning is truly a sport for sadists.

Out of Bounds

Ahhh, the basketball court. Yet another no-woman zone. I guess that's not entirely true. I have seen the occasional female on the court. But she's always Olympic-level amazing, three-point shots tossed off with ease. Whereas if I was to ever step onto the court, it would be for the sole task of handing out water bottles and towels.

See, time on the basketball court is coveted, competitive, cutthroat. There isn't room for amateurs. This is where dudes go to blow off steam and regress to the days of playground shoving matches and name calling. And if you've ever stood on the sidelines and watched a game in progress, you know how rough it can get. There's always a fight on the verge of breaking out. On the court, there's a fine line between competitive and combative. It doesn't matter what time of day you go, there's always some type of screaming match in progress.

So, in my opinion, unless you're there to watch, it's best to just keep on walking. The basketball court is tough, and the players are mean. Personally, I'd feel safer spending a night in the mosh pit at a punk show. But hey, that's just me.

Yoga + Bad Lighting = Non-maste

Why the hell do gyms think they can teach yoga? Everything about the gym (the lighting, the noise, the meatheads) is the polar opposite of a calming "yoga experience." When you take a yoga class, you should have no outside distractions interfering with your experience. And as someone who is easily distracted by everything—from a car alarm to a nearby nose whistler—silence is essential. That said, my friend Lizzie, who loves the yoga class at her gym, insisted her class would be distraction free. The teacher, she claimed, was amazing and skilled at keeping her class focused. Either Lizzie was the biggest smack talker in town, or this class was worth checking out. I decided to stop by and find out for myself.

The teacher, as promised, was warm, lovely, and seemed at ease slipping herself into a pretzel position while standing on one leg. And, I have to admit, the class was overall quite enjoyable, were it not for the Venice Beach muscle heads lifting weights three feet away. While I couldn't hear their grunts of pain or their encouraging shouts to "feel the burn," I could still see their faces, their expressions, their cheesy high fives. They were, after all, only a thin sheet of Plexiglas away. Not to mention that anytime someone got up to use the restroom, they would open the door, allowing the throbbing club music to seep in. So it didn't matter how great the teacher was. She could've been the Maharishi, but having to compete against the music, the semidistant sounds of shouting, and the laboratory lighting, the deck was stacked against her. It wasn't a fair fight. And, as expected, the gym, the eternal bully, won again.

My Girl Wants to Pilates All the Time

Pilates is the lazy man's exercise. So it's hard for me to say with any real conviction that I hate it. I mean, what's to hate? You lie on a mat, hold your legs in the air, and take it easy. You could even get a few winks in if you wanted. I mean, I guess it can be strenuous from time to time, and sometimes even leave you with that satisfying sore feeling. But more often than not, when I take a Pilates class, I don't even break a sweat.

Although, it should be noted that my Pilates teacher has an amazing body. From behind, you'd think she was in her twenties when in reality she's probably pushing late forties. (Forgive me, Tanis.) But does that mean it's the only thing she does to maintain her slamming body? I doubt it. She probably lives on a diet of tasteless twigs and exercises from dawn to dusk. And yet everyone thinks it's the Pilates.

So while I always recommend Pilates to gym haters, has it really changed my body significantly? I don't think so. Unless holding your arms in the air for over a minute counts as something. And I don't think it does. I say, better to just sleep in.

The Players

The Show-Off: She's the one who knows all the moves and looks hot doing them. She wears perfect workout clothes, and looks even hotter when she sweats. She is your classic nemesis . . . because she's perfect and she knows it.
Your Goal: To witness her lose her balance and fall off her stationary bike. A girl can dream, can't she?

The Righteous Farter: He's the guy who will shamelessly rip one in the middle of a downward dog. He's not one to let a little gas get in the way of his exercise. Unfortunately, if you're anywhere in the vicinity, it'll become your problem.
Your Goal: Sidestep the gasbag.

The Grunter: He's the guy who is working out and wants everyone to know it. Look, buddy, we're all putting our time in at the gym. We're hurting too. But why do we need to be subjected to your grunts of pain? Put a muzzle on it.
Your Goal: Plug in, and tune out.

Class Etiquette

- Avoid the front row.
- Bring enough water to hydrate a village.
- Brace yourself for pain.
- Don't pass gas in class.
- Don't strike up a conversation in the middle of a session.

Class Survival Techniques

Boot camp is the basic training of the exercise world. The best way to survive is to stretch beforehand, practice your ducking skills, and bring water—lots and lots of water.

Spinning is for people who are serious about working out. This is definitely not a beginner's class. So rookies, stick to the back row, out of the instructor's line of sight, and just try to keep up.

Oh yeah, and bring an extra shirt. You will be soaked in your own stink.

Yoga—the best way to enjoy it is to keep the distractions to a minimum. Avoid sitting near the older gentleman in the loose shorts. And, above all, if you want to avoid the vapors, commence mouth breathing immediately.

Pilates is mostly spent prone on the mat. So if you enjoy this kind of activity, then cough up the dough and invest in your own mat. Things can get pretty smelly when you're sharing.

Basketball is the only place where adults are allowed to act like kids. Tantrums run rampant, emotions are at an all-time high, and attitude on the court is kicking. So run with the wolves and do whatever it takes to survive.

CHAPTER ELEVEN

THE POOL:

TO SWIM OR SNOT TO SWIM

To put it bluntly, the pool is a germaphobe's worst nightmare. It's a cesspool of snot, a watering hole of hairballs, a bog of Band-Aids, all tossed together with the inexplicable warm spot. Which leads one to ask: Could adults really be peeing in the pool? Aren't we a little old for that kind of behavior? But alas, that isn't the only problem. Gym swimming pools tend to be small, cramped spaces, which make lane sharing an acrobatic, aquatic dance that would confound even Esther Williams. Not to mention, the pool is chock full of reckless swimmers (the drifters, show-offs, and flailers), old people pruning, (the ladder chatters), and inappropriate lifeguards who think that a pair of red shorts and a whistle make them king of the water world. So next time you take the plunge, prepare yourself for the aqua assault.

Maintain Your Lane

One of the most important things about the pool is to know what level swimmer you are. Are you a slow swimmer or a speedy swimmer? Are you only fast for two laps, or are your splits Olympic level? Do you cramp up after twenty minutes, or is your next goal to swim the English Channel? Is the doggie paddle your preferred stroke, or are you a flip-turning freestyle machine? Whatever your swimming ability, it's essential to use the correct lane. A tailgating fast swimmer or a road-blocking slowpoke can really screw up a workout and make for an extremely frustrating half hour in the pool. So don't be afraid to narc on a sluggish lane mate or demand an aisle change for Mark Spitz. Remember, this is your pool too, dammit.

Here's a tip: Think of the pool as a four-lane highway. Each lane has a certain speed: slow, medium slow, medium fast, fast. Find the speed that best suits you and stay there. Don't get cocky and change lanes after a few laps, unless you know you can keep up with the speed demons.

Whether it's the Sloppy Swimmer or the Lane Log, an unwanted pool mate can strike at any turn. One of the biggest pet peeves for the pool regular is the Drifter. Lost in their own world, Drifters crash into other people, swim into the lane lines, and jab unsuspecting swimmers without apology. This is the reason they paint thick black lines on the bottom of the pool, people. Open your eyes.

Next on the list of annoying obstacles is the Flailer. These are the folks who seem to have no apparent control of their limbs. They flop. They splash. They flail. In fact, they look like they could drown at any moment, which forces swimmers to modify their workout or risk a mouthful of pool water. Flailers are like fussy children. They disrupt everyone and everything and are virtually impossible to ignore. If only they could tone it down and master the mechanics of their stroke, which is usually freestyle, then they wouldn't fall into the category of yet another swimmer who clearly doesn't understand pool etiquette. People come to exercise, not to dodge psychotic swimmers trying to stay afloat. Just remember: When it comes to freestyle, less is more—less flailing, more gliding.

Another great pool offense is when the crappy swimmer insists on starting his workout with a rousing lap or two of the butterfly. This arrogant display inevitably leads to half of the pool's water emptying onto the floor, leaving a trail of irritated pool patrons in the pompous swimmer's wake.

The butterfly stroker often tends to be male. And his choice of stroke is crucial in understanding just who he is and what makes him tick. He's basically your classic show-off—he likes to make a big splash. And nothing does that better than the butterfly. It's a complicated stroke that requires tremendous coordination and strength. Thankfully, it's nearly impossible for an amateur to do more than two laps, so it'll end as quickly as it began. The "butterfliers" are the pre-ejaculators of the pool: all talk, no timing. Not literally, of course. Because that would just be gross.

And then there is the backstroker, another oblivious offender. Paddling backwards, they have no idea where they're going, where they're headed, and where the pool ends. This inevitably leads to a collision and possibly a bruise. So if you see a backstroker lumbering toward you, duck out of the way or prepare to be poked. They are the Mister Magoos of the water world.

And, of course, how could we forget about the breaststroker, the docile turtles of the pool? While they're a better, more conscientious, breed of swimmer—they keep their eyes open, heads up, and hair dry—they are also known for their frog kicks, which can cause unsightly bruises if you don't stay out of their way. So, keep your eyes open and reflexes alert. Just because they move at a snail's pace doesn't mean they don't pack a punch.

Finally, there's the Lane Log. These buoyant buoys tend to be belligerent old people. Both male and female, they like to linger at the ladders, soak at the end of lanes, and complain about everything. The water is never warm enough. The music is too harsh on the ears. The tiles are too slippery—someone could fall and break a hip. And their favorite pastime is bothering the lifeguards about their lane placement. Oh yeah, that's another thing, Lane Logs have a tremendous sense of entitlement. And nothing gets their goat more than being told that their half-hour time limit has expired. Fortunately, they are easy to avoid—just keep your head underwater, and go about your workout. Unless you're a lifeguard . . . Then, good luck. I recommend earplugs.

Avoid the Warm Spot

Traditionally, the warm spot is something you might encounter in a kiddie pool. That said, they've been known to crop up in more adult settings, i.e., the lap pool. I'm not a fan of laying blame or pointing fingers, but in this case I will. I have two words for you: old folks. Now, I'm not making a blanket accusation here. All I'm saying is that the pool is always dotted with patches of warm water after an aqua aerobics class. So watch out for the slow-moving seniors, and always shower after a swim.

The Floater

It's gross to think of the pool as a giant germ bog, but sadly, it's true. Sure, the management asks you to take a shower before entering the pool, but are people really washing with soap? Or are they just barely rinsing off the dirt? Who knows; either way, the next stop for them is the pool, another giant bathtub. And then it's chlorine to the rescue. I'd say thank god for the intense chlorination. But talk to any diehard swimmer and they'll tell you stories of green hair and bloodshot eyes.

Not to mention the pool is chock full of schmutz. Not literally, of course. But most swimmers have encountered their fair share of lost Band-Aids, loose hairs, and booger blobs. So what do you do when you discover one of these pool staples up ahead? Five words: deep breaths and quick kicking. Or bravely lift the offending item out of the pool and consider it your good deed for the day.

Crossing the Bikini Line

Since the pool is not really considered a trip to the beach, the well-maintained bikini line is strongly encouraged but not mandatory. In fact, most competitive swimwear is, well . . . quite forgiving. The bathing suits are cut so conservatively that they could be mistaken for overalls. In other words, if you haven't been able to get to your waxer in a while, fear not. All your Speedo requires is a little tucking action and you'll be ready to take the plunge. However, if you're looking for an excuse to take the night off, an unruly bikini line can work in your favor. If you're a stickler for smoothness, consider the visible line a deal breaker, leaving you free from gym duty until you've taken a dip in hot wax. If hairiness is not a particular concern of yours, and the pool is your underwater refuge, then an overgrown bush can serve as an excellent deterrent to unwanted advances and impromptu conversations. Just flash the unkempt hairline and watch as conversations come to a screeching halt.

That said, there is nothing more annoying than women who wear their good bikinis to work out. This isn't Club Med. This is the crusty indoor pool at the Y. We're not here to pick up men. And we're not here to wait while the bikini babes try to figure out how to artfully remove their wedgies every two laps. So down with the cute suits. Save it for the beach, ladies.

But perhaps even more offensive than the bikini wearer is the person who allows their suit to get so old (which, by the way, doesn't take long, with the toxic chlorine eating away at it) that the suit loses all of its elasticity and becomes see-through. In short, there's a peep show going on and it's of *your ass*. So monitor the erosion of the nylon or you may find yourself wearing only your birthday suit.

The Players

The Geezers: They hug the walls. They block the ladders. They complain to the lifeguard. And they hog the lanes with their slow-moving kickboards. Basically, they're a thorn in your side, a pesky presence, a wrinkly roadblock. So just swim around them and don't get sucked in.

Your Goal: Dodge the Lane Log.

The Splashers: They're the sloppy swimmers who like to make a big, dramatic entrance. The best advice I can give is to move out of their way and try not to scrape your knuckles. Things can get messy with a Splasher around.

Your Goal: Don't swallow too much water.

Swimming Pool Etiquette

- Don't wear two past-their-prime bathing suits on top of each other. In this case, two isn't better than one.
- Don't wear a Speedo unless you're a serious swimmer . . . or a European who doesn't know any better.
- Don't forget to wear your bathing cap in the pool. Be part of the solution, not the problem. Stop the stray-hair syndrome.
- Don't hang out at the pool. It's for swimming, not lounging.
- Don't linger on the ladder and chatter.
- Don't hug the sides. If you aren't comfortable letting go of the edge, why the hell are you in the pool?

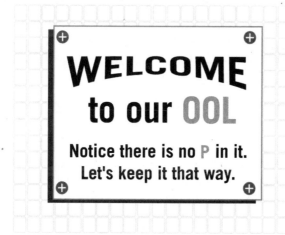

WELCOME to our OOL

Notice there is no P in it.
Let's keep it that way.

CHAPTER TWELVE

THE JUICE BAR:
WHEATGRASS, ENEMY OF THE PEOPLE

The juice bar is one of the more recent gym inventions. Actually, it's not really an invention. It's more of a money-scheming concoction—you can exercise and pay to rehydrate all in one place. It's the classic gym fixture that screams Los Angeles, even though the first one I saw was in New York in the early nineties. The juice bar serves as the perfect refueling station for that calorie-conscious, on-the-go individual—or so the gym management wants you to think. In fact, they'd be happy if you spent all of your free time at the gym. And if they can provide you with a tasteless smoothie, vitamin-rich PowerBar, or faux healthy sandwich, they are one step closer to sucking you in to gym acceptance.

You see, it all starts innocently enough. One day, you arrive at the gym and realize you forgot your water, so you head over to the juice bar to purchase a bottle. And that's when you discover they also serve fresh fruit smoothies. Mmmm, your favorite. So you order one. Then the next time you're heading for the treadmill, you find yourself craving another. Now you're going to the gym more frequently, and always with extra change in your pocket. And you realize one day as you mindlessly march over to the juice bar that you no longer have control of your thoughts, your actions, and even worse, you've gone from a gym hater to a gym regular. In other words, you have officially crossed over to gym cult member status. If you don't believe that this exists, just sit back and watch as seemingly normal people suck back "healthy" refreshments and then rebound back into the gym for another round on the StairMaster. Or perhaps the juice bar is just another way for the gym to extract more money from you. In addition to the expensive gym membership you recently purchased, they're now after the money in your wallet, too. Either way, this cycle of member mistreatment must end.

And it doesn't stop there. The juice bar is one thing in a long list of "added luxuries" the gym now offers. They range from the café to the hot tub, and for some folks, the bonus features are what the gym is all about. They may join because of the sauna and stay for the fruit smoothie. Whereas, a glass of juice and the opportunity to sit in a hot tub with strangers is the last thing in the world I'm interested in doing. And it's not just because the thought of communal hot tubs gives me a rash. It is simply that, for me, the gym is a place to exercise, interact with as few people as possible, and then bolt the moment I've finished my last sit-up. So try as I may, I can't understand why anyone would want to prolong their stay at the gym. Is sipping an overly complicated, utterly tasteless fruit juice really worth hanging out after hours? Let's be honest here: Unless you are bovine in nature, it would be a lie to say you genuinely enjoy the taste of wheatgrass.

As far as I can tell, the juice bar is the dividing line, the place that separates the gym-goer from the gym lover. The goer enters the gym with great reluctance, while the gym lover relishes his or her time at the gym. Even if I was starving, light-headed, and wobbly kneed, I wouldn't stop to have a crappy, frozen, fruity beverage. No, thank you. I save all of my dining and drinking pleasures for off-campus pursuits. So if you're anything like me, it's important to get in and get out. The juice isn't going to be good, and the company will be even worse. Now, if these issues plague your daily journey to the gym, then read on and learn how to stop the juice abuse.

The Gym as Social Destination

For many people (none of whom I am friends with), the gym is a social haven, a destination, a place to meet up and hang out. These people have friends who work at the gym, trainers they spend time with, equipment they lounge on, and Jacuzzis they prune in. In short, they have no life. The gym is their life.

I spoke to a trainer who told me that, aside from the actual training aspect, he considers being a therapist part of his job. For roughly half of his clients, he is their only human contact during the day. Either they're stay-at-home moms, housewives, or freaky shut-ins. And the trainer's role is elevated to adviser, motivator, and friend. Now what does that say about people who are willing to share their most intimate secrets with their trainers? One, that they should get out more. Two, that they should get some more friends (preferably friends who aren't on the payroll). And three, that they should really stop sharing secrets with their trainers. Wake up, people. The gym isn't for hanging out; it's for working out. If you want additional stimuli, go to a museum, meet a friend for lunch, treat yourself to a movie, take a hike—*anything*, really. Just try to refrain from confiding in your trainer. He's just going to turn around and tell someone else about your problems. How do you think I know so much?

Vitamin Violators

If you are purchasing your vitamins, protein powders, or muscle enhancers at the gym, you are doing it at the wrong place. Whatever you're buying, put it down. Go to a health food store and find a knowledgeable clerk, someone who really knows what they're selling, as opposed to some steroid freak with bulging veins. You want to know about the health benefits and risks (mainly risks) of taking vitamins that promise muscle definition and slimmer waistlines. Because as much as I wish a trim, svelte figure could be purchased in pill form, I can't help but be dubious. And you don't want to have a heart attack at thirty. So put down the vanilla-flavored crack powder and head for the exit.

The Players

The Trainers: For most trainers, the juice bar is their faculty lounge. It's where they go to unwind and refuel. Usually they can be found consuming something protein rich and calorie light that often resembles an old slipper. And chances are, this oversize muscle head finds his dry tofu slab just as flavorless as it looks.

Your Goal: Don't stand too close. You might be mistaken for a tasty treat.

The Bored and Jobless: They come in all different shades, shapes, and sizes. They are the housewives killing time, the actors awaiting their next audition, and the dilettantes in search of companionship and attention. Usually this gang of assorted misfits can be found in the company of trainers, or one another. So avoid them at all costs, or prepare to pay in boredom.

Your Goal: Dodge the eager beavers swapping headshots and nail polish.

Juice Bar Etiquette

- Don't settle for a sandwich. Expand your horizons.
- Don't eat food that has been prepared next to sweat.
- Bring a book. Never leave yourself open.
- Wear large sunglasses. Create the illusion of being an unapproachable celebrity.

CHAPTER THIRTEEN

THE WARM DOWN:
EXPOSING POSES

The best part of any trip to the gym is being done, finished, free. It's like getting out of work early. Or a really boring class on a gorgeous day. You've done your time. You've worked hard. You've sweated in public. And you even have the cherry-red face to prove it. So now it's time to mosey on down to the stretching area for some well-deserved, low-impact stretching. The only problem is, the room is crowded, people are chatting, and you're so sweaty, you don't know what to do with yourself. Not to mention, there's a creepy dude in the corner scoping out your booty. So how do you maneuver this minefield?

Silence Is Golden
Now, I don't know about your gym, but when you walk into the

stretching area at mine, the first thing you see is a giant sign that reads, SHHHH! QUIET AREA. It even has a little illustration of a mime making a shushing face. So that should really tell you this isn't the right place to strike up a conversation with your friend about shoes, or that hot date you had with a college freshman last night. The stretching area should command the same respect as a movie theater—pretend the movie is in progress, and shut the hell up.

But even worse than the "babblers" are the people who insist on doing yoga next to you. It goes a little something like this: up, down, grunt. Up, down, grunt. They groan, they moan, they breathe loudly. It's enough to make you want to punch them in the face. I mean, come on, this is the stretching area, a place to cool down, to unwind. So if you want to brush up on your yoga, take a class. Or do it at home. But please don't practice "breath of fire" next to me. It's distracting, loud, and often causes spitting. And that's just plain disgusting.

The Crotch Sweat Blues

In my experience, exposing a sweaty crotch is a mistake you'll only make once. Let me set the scene for you. You're wearing light gray stretch pants and you've just finished working out. So you head to the mats for some stretching. But when you bend over, legs apart, you discover a giant swath of crotch sweat that slightly resembles a Rorschach test. And as you discretely close your legs and pretend that nothing happened, you vow to yourself that you will *never* ever wear anything tight or light in color when sweat is involved.

Now, when I go to the gym, I wear one color and one color only: black. Black both hides sweat and is the color of mourning, which is appropriate given that working out is a somber, joyless occasion. So when it comes to high-impact workouts, put away your light-colored shorts and stretch pants. There is nothing worse than letting the world know that you have a sweaty crotch.

Triple-X Stretches

Is there a stretch you just won't do? Something that is vaguely pornographic, borderline gynecological, something involving legs akimbo that makes you feel like a dirty dimestore whore? Well, trust me when I say this: You're not alone. Too many of my friends complain of creepy men with wandering eyes that drive them to stretch in the privacy of their own homes.

I once made the mistake of trying out a hip stretch my trainer had shown me on the mats, when I should have saved it for my living room. It looks a little something like this: me on my back, legs spread eagle, arms in crotch. I wish I could be the bigger person and rise above the obscenity of it all. But the truth is, it just isn't relaxing knowing that butt hounds and crotch watchers are watching your every move. Consequently, my hips are tight and I can't do anything about it. So, thanks a lot, pervs. Hope you got a nice look, because next time I'll be sure to wear my light gray pants and then you can feast your eyes on a sweaty crotch. Ah, revenge. They say it's a dish served cold and sweaty.

The Players

The Conceited Breathers: These are the smug people who profess the virtues of deep breathing. They take themselves beyond seriously, with their closed eyes and fake peacefulness. They're part of the culture of indulgence. I only wish they would save it for Lamaze class.

Your Goal: To breathe longer and louder. Two can play at that game.

The Grunters and the Moaners: The name says it all. These are the men and women (although they're mostly men) whose every move is accompanied by a deep moan or a pained grunt. For them, stretching is akin to torture, and touching their toes is sheer hell. They should be put in solitary confinement for noise violation.

Your Goal: To stand far, far away.

The Entitled Talkers: These are the loudmouths that blabber shamelessly as if the entire room were interested in their lives. They're obnoxious and, even worse, impervious to criticism. You can tell them to be quiet, but don't expect them to react or care.

Your Goal: Block the talk by humming. Loudly.

The Sweaty Mess: This is the pile of perspiration hyperventilating in the corner. Chances are, they haven't been to the gym in a while and have just pushed themselves to the limit in an effort to make up for lost time or lapsed membership. They won't bother you—although keep your eyes open for projectile sweat. They know not what they do.

Your Goal: To not slip in the sweat.

The Flock of Jocks: This is the herd of sweaty guys who work out together, party together, and have repressed homosexual fantasies together. Easy to spot, they're the ones dressed in head-to-toe sports or fraternity gear. Don't get too close . . . their conversation is sure to offend the sensibilities and burn the ears.

Your Goal: To remind yourself that high school is long over. Now, breathe a sigh of relief.

The Lurker: This is the man whose most distinguishing characteristic is the amount of time he spends in the stretching area. He stretches, stares, and then pretends to stretch some more. He won't come up to you, he'll just stare. Which, actually, may be creepier.

Your Goal: To step out of his line of vision. And to never show him your rootin' tootin' booty.

Stretching Area Etiquette

- Don't hog the balls.
- Don't do extreme lunges in short-shorts.
- X marks the mat. Don't leave a sweat mark for someone else to clean up.
- Don't pose in front of the mirrors.
- Don't chitchat with your neighbor.
- Don't groan loudly.
- Don't involve everyone in your workout.
- Always make it quick.

CHAPTER FOURTEEN

TIME TO DO IT

ALL OVER AGAIN

The downside of successfully completing a workout is that tomorrow—or, more likely, the day after that—you'll be heading back to the gym. Again.

Exercise is a responsibility that comes with age. As adults, it's our job to stay in shape and keep the dreaded osteoporosis at bay. We can no longer rely on pushy PE teachers, school requirements, and team sports. Now it's up to us. And it sucks. Not only do we have to watch what we eat (i.e., no more midnight McDonald's drive-through pit stops), it's our job to remain active, in shape, and looking good. Motivations may differ. For example, I go to the gym so that my husband, Dave, doesn't wake up one day to find a hideously misshapen blob sleeping next to him; while Dave exercises because his doctor told him that he has the cholesterol level of a ninety-year-old

man. So whatever the reason, I regret to report that gym attendance is required.

When It's Time to Say No

All of that said, there are times in one's life when it is possible to
"over gym." It's like going overboard on a diet. You start out with
innocent intentions. Perhaps there is a dress you want to fit into,
a pair of pants that aren't quite closing, or a Buddha belly that
has been getting in the way. Next thing you know, you're weighing your food and calorie counting. You don't want to be one of
those people. They have bad breath and no sense of humor.

Going to the gym can be just as addictive as a fad diet. It
works the same way, and it's easy to lose control. Before I got
married, in a mad attempt to be skinny, toned, and devastat-
ingly hot, I went to the gym every day. And the next thing I
knew, I had become one of those women I like to mock and
ridicule. Now, before you lose all respect for me, once the wedding was over, I snapped back to my normal, gym-hating,
exercise-avoiding self. And frankly, I like me better that way.
That's why it's important to go easy on the attendance and
never beat yourself up if you don't feel up to going. The gym
changes people—don't let that happen to you.

Am I Strong Enough, Handsome Enough, Tan Enough?

And, most importantly, do not, I repeat, do not fall into the
trap of feeling inadequate just because you don't look like

Jennifer Aniston or Brad Pitt. Most movie stars devote their entire lives to staying thin and in shape. What you may not realize is that actresses work out like mental patients. They spend whole mornings in sessions with trainers, and are often on strict, no-fun, no-booze diets, which means they are always hungry . . . and sober.

The point is, if you need to look unnaturally hot, you know what to do. Otherwise, have a long-term plan in effect. Denying yourself on a regular basis is no way to live. You want to be able to dine with friends, eat the occasional wedge of Brie, and share bottles of wine. So be grateful that you aren't an actor, and order some dessert. You're still going to have to pay for it on the treadmill, so what the hell, go crazy.

Acknowledgments

This book could never have been written without the insight, embarrassing episodes, and utterly humiliating moments of many people. They know who they are. But what the hell, why not name them: Aaron, Amanda, Ari, Chris, Dawn, Eric, Erin, Gigi, Jason, Jesse, Jonathan, Kristen, Linda, Lizzie, Melissa, Mike, Olivia, Rebecca, Ross, Saskia, Sebastian, Todd, and Trish. Thank you for sharing and making your pain my fodder. And, of course, to my parents, Susan and Howard, for all of their love and support. Finally, to Trish, my wonderful friend and amazing editor, for helping me see the light at the end of the tunnel.

Jessica Kaminsky currently has four memberships to health clubs, two personal trainers, and still would rather give up bread for a week than go to the gym for even an hour. She lives in Los Angeles with her sympathetic husband.